THE KID'S USER GUIDE TO A
HUMAN LIFE

THE KID'S USER GUIDE TO A

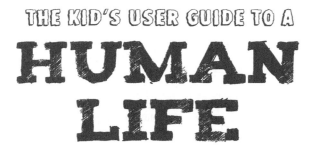

HUMAN LIFE

BOOK ONE: AN OPEN MIND

REBECCA BRENNER

NEW YORK

THE KID'S USER GUIDE TO A **HUMAN LIFE**
BOOK ONE: AN OPEN MIND

© 2014 **REBECCA BRENNER**. Illustrated by **BROOKE KEMMERER**.

Published in New York, New York, by Morgan James Publishing. Morgan James and The Entrepreneurial Publisher are trademarks of Morgan James, LLC. www.MorganJamesPublishing.com

The Morgan James Speakers Group can bring authors to your live event. For more information or to book an event visit The Morgan James Speakers Group at www.TheMorganJamesSpeakersGroup.com.

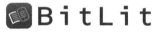

A FREE eBook edition is available
with the purchase of this print book

CLEARLY PRINT YOUR NAME IN THE BOX ABOVE

Instructions to claim your free eBook edition:
1. Download the BitLit app for Android or iOS
2. Write your name in UPPER CASE in the box
3. Use the BitLit app to submit a photo
4. Download your eBook to any device

ISBN 978-1-61448-923-8 paperback
ISBN 978-1-61448-924-5 eBook
ISBN 978-1-61448-925-2 audio
Library of Congress Control Number:
2013951452

Cover Design by:
Chris Treccani
www.3dogdesign.net

Interior Design by:
Bonnie Bushman
bonnie@caboodlegraphics.com

In an effort to support local communities, raise awareness and funds, Morgan James Publishing donates a percentage of all book sales for the life of each book to Habitat for Humanity Peninsula and Greater Williamsburg.

Get involved today, visit
www.MorganJamesBuilds.com.

Habitat
for Humanity®
Peninsula and
Greater Williamsburg
Building Partner

For Brenner and Emerson —
thank you for waking me up
—RB

For Stella and Locke
—BK

INTRODUCTION

*"O Nobly Born, O you of glorious origins, remember
your radiant true nature, the essence of Mind. Trust it.
Return to it. It is home."*

—Tibetan Book of the Dead

Y ou are magnificent. An Adventurer of epic proportions—born into this wild adventure called Life. This adventure is rich—full of great joy, unbreakable bonds, and unspeakable wonderment. However, it is important to know right from the start that this adventure will also present you with challenges, disappointments, and loss. There is nothing you can do to change this. It is an intricate part of your journey. When you encounter these challenges, know it is not a reflection of who you truly are. It is just how this adventure of Life goes.

For your Life is dynamic—always shifting and changing. Once you think you see the path ahead of you, it will shift and change right before your eyes. This ever-changing path is also an intricate part of your journey. Any Great Adventurer knows to stay agile in body and mind—and you are a Great Adventurer.

This Life is even quite mysterious at times, with many unknowns. But you, Adventurer, were born brave and courageous. Know that sometimes it will even take monumental bravery and courage not to lose your wits as Life shifts and changes around you. For even when you forget your own bravery and courage, know that they are always within you, Adventurous One!

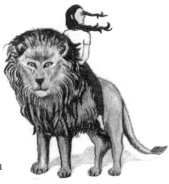

All Adventurers need special tools to brave the unknown journey of Life—through your

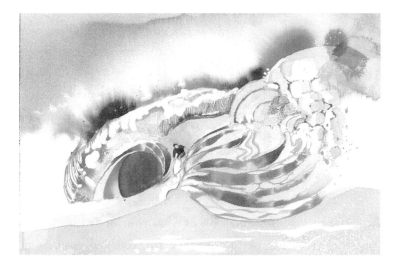

greatest joys as well as your greatest challenges. Do not worry. You were born with all the tools you need. You may travel far into the world seeking special tools for your journey, but know what you need is already within you. Remember this—you are not lacking in anything you need for this journey. You came into this Life whole. Even though your tools are countless, your most prized tools are your Vehicle, your Compass, and your Inner Navigator.

Your Vehicle is your miraculous body. Your lovely beating heart, pumping beautiful blood to the edges of your skin and back again. Your gracefully breathing lungs, circulating and recycling breath through each microscopically tiny cell in your body. Your vital organs and digestive system working harmoniously with the healthy foods you eat and clean water you drink. Your arms and legs moving you along your adventure—pulling in close all that you love and letting go of what you no longer need. Your muscles, ligaments,

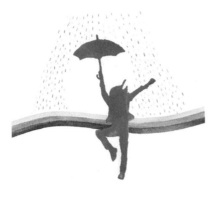

and tendons allow you to move effortlessly along your path. With your senses—touch, taste, smell, hearing, and sight—you are able to explore every nook and cranny that sparks your interest.

And this is just a small bit of what your body can do! You certainly have the perfect Vehicle for your adventure—no matter what size, shape, or color. It is uniquely yours, Great Adventurer, made especially for you!

Your Compass is your lively emotions. Your emotions give you feedback as to whether you are on the right path and where you may need to grow, shift, or change. Emotions such as anxiety and fear, when used mindfully, will alert you to treacherous conditions and experiences along your journey. Emotions such as anger and

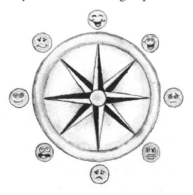

frustration, when matched with wisdom, will help you to create healthy boundaries that nudge you in the right direction.

Do not fear your big emotions, they truly are part of your inner guide. With mindfulness, this inner guide will lead you safely through the foggy parts of your adventure.

Your ceaselessly amazing mind is your Inner Navigator—steering you through clear skies as well as rough passages. Your Inner Navigator's original nature is that of an Open Mind and its default setting is one of a Chattering Mind. How you use your Open Mind and Chattering Mind will greatly determine how you experience your journey. For the content of your Chattering Mind deeply influences how well your Vehicle and Compass work. Your Inner Navigator—when left unchecked—can wreak havoc on your other tools creating struggle and strife through your entire being.

For this reason, let's begin this adventure by looking deeply into how your Inner Navigator works. When you understand your own mind, you will learn who you truly are and getting to know yourself may be the grandest part of your adventure!

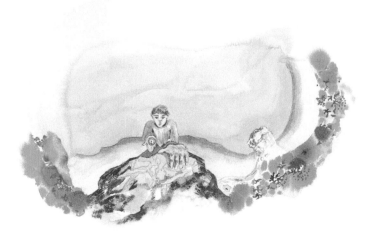

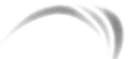

CHAPTER 1

"The intuitive mind is a sacred gift and the rational mind is a faithful servant. We have created a society that honors the servant and has forgotten the gift."

–Albert Einstein

Your brain may just be the most important tool you carry with you through this adventurous Life. It controls ALL of your Vehicle's functions, affects your Compass and Inner Navigator, and stores all of your memories, likes, and dislikes. Because your brain is so complex, knowing how to use it can seem perplexing at first. But once you know your own brain a little better it will be your best ally as you journey through Life.

Let's take a closer look. On the surface, most everyone's brain is created equally with all the same parts.

All these parts do essentially the same thing in every brain. The cerebrum controls voluntary movement, speech,

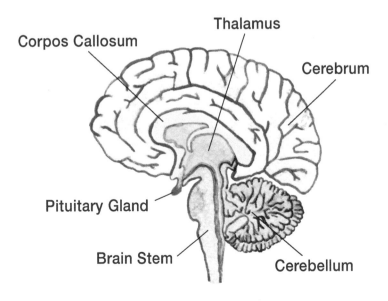

and memory. The thalamus regulates information coming in from your senses. The cerebellum helps to coordinate your movements, balance and equilibrium. The pituitary gland controls your hormones and functions in your body like blood pressure and body temperature. And the brain stem regulates your breathing.

Brains are divided into two sections—the right and left hemispheres—with a band of nerve fibers down the middle called the corpus callosum. The corpus callosum connects the two hemispheres, allowing them to communicate with one another. And each hemisphere is responsible for different experiences, skills, and behaviors.

Even though everyone's brain has essentially the same parts, the way these parts relate to each other is different for

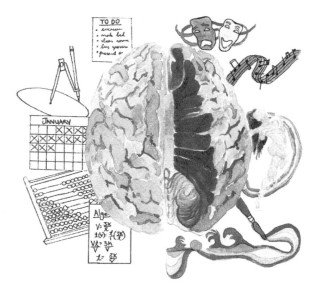

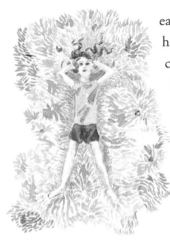

each person. How your brain is hardwired is unique to you—creating a one-of-a-kind Inner Navigator. That means that no one who has ever lived or will live can see the world just as you do. Nor can you truly see the world as someone else does.

On a physical level, your brain is hardwired by billions of neurons and the pathways they create throughout your brain called neuron pathways. Your brain takes in information from all around you to inform the neurons on which pathways to create. Your family interactions and dynamics, the community you live in, your friendships, your schooling, the music you listen to, the books you read, the television shows you watch all create pathways in your brain. All the information you take in from the world around you and how you process it create your neuron pathways, which in many ways make you You!

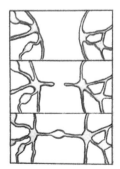

If you pay attention, you can hear this "You" chattering away all day long between your

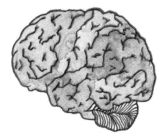

ears. Your neuron pathways come alive with a voice that is so constant that you may not have even noticed it going on and on and on and on. Here, take five minutes to sit quietly and listen. Close your eyes and pay attention to what you say to yourself.

Can you hear it—your mind chattering away? When left to its own devices your mind chatters away all day, influencing everything you do and feel. This chatter is based on all of your past, learned, and inherited experiences. The neuron pathways in your brain were created by your greatest successes and your most challenging moments.

In all the endless possibilities that are available in every moment, your chatter stays focused on a small set of experiences, looping through them continuously and filtering everything you do through this small set of experiences. Your Chattering Mind does this mainly to keep your Vehicle safe, help you along your path effectively and efficiently, and move you towards what your Compass finds pleasurable. The Chattering Mind also keeps you from having to learn the same things over and over again.

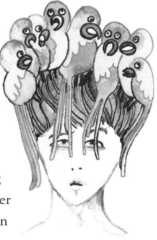

What happens most times, though, is that your Chattering Mind takes over your Inner Attention and moves you into an automatic and unconscious way of being. Because the Chattering Mind uses only your past experiences to steer you towards safety, when left unchecked, it covers over your ability to see the present moment clearly. This limits the natural openness of your true Adventurous Self. And this in turn limits your experience of the magic of your Life unfolding moment by moment.

CHAPTER 2

*"Your body is precious. It is your vehicle for awakening.
Treat it with care."*

—Buddha

Your brain is part of a larger system in the body called the nervous system. Your nervous system is an amazing and intricate communication network between your Vehicle, Compass, and Inner Navigator. It is divided into the central nervous system and peripheral nervous system.

Your central nervous system includes the brain and spinal column. Your peripheral nervous system includes the somatic nervous system (bundle of nerve fibers) and autonomic nervous system. And the autonomic nervous system is divided into three parts: the sympathetic nervous system, the parasympathetic nervous system, and the entric nervous system.

Different parts of your body can communicate with one another through your nervous system to keep you balanced and to keep your Vehicle working smoothly. Your involuntary movements like blinking and breathing are regulated by your nervous system. This automatic movement of certain body parts frees up some of your focus. Can you imagine having to blink your eyes, breathe your lungs, and beat your own heart? Larger, voluntary movements like walking, running, and jumping are also processed through your nervous system. Really, everything you do registers through your entire nervous system.

Your nervous system is always trying to keep you safe. Take, for example, when your fingers get too close to an open flame. Your skin feels heat, which then sends information along your nerves and nervous system to your brain, which in turn sends information back to your muscles to move your fingers away from the flame. All of this communication happens in seconds! Your nervous system works non-stop to keep you healthy and well.

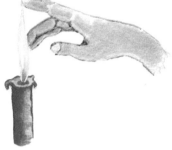

When all is going smoothly your nervous system mainly runs on the parasympathetic nervous system. This is sometimes referred to as the "rest and digest" nervous system because that is the exact message it is sending to your entire body. When your Compass is registering feelings of happiness and health your parasympathetic nervous system restores the body's energy by lowering your heart rate and blood pressure, sending blood to your digestive system, and helping the diaphragm create slow, deep breaths. Your Vehicle, in turn, sends this feel-good information to the Inner Navigator, which allows your Chattering Mind to relax and open.

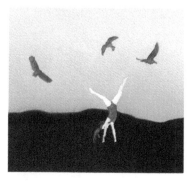

Close your eyes for a moment and remember the last time you felt happy and carefree. How did your body feel? Were you relaxed? Did you feel peaceful?

Ideally, you will spend the majority of your adventure with your body resting in the parasympathetic nervous system and your mind relaxed. This would give you all the energy you need to play, create, be present to the beauty of the natural world, and enjoy your loved ones. You were meant to live in a state of balance, health, and joy. In fact, your Vehicle is always working towards this state of health. No matter what you feed it, how you treat it, or how much sleep you get, your body is always trying its best to keep you in a healthy and balanced state. Of course, a body that is being treated unkindly can only do so much!

However, when there is any threat of danger, your body quickly switches into the sympathetic nervous system, also referred to as the "flight or fight" nervous system. When your Compass registers feelings of stress or threat, the sympathetic nervous system prepares your body for flight (fleeing from danger) or fight (protecting yourself) by gathering all of your body's energy for alertness and action. In these moments, the sympathetic nervous system increases your heart rate and blood pressure, slows digestion, and quickens and shortens your breath. This quick boost of energy helps you swiftly get to safety.

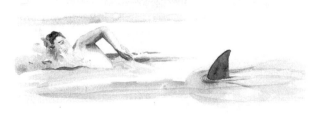

But stress signals are not always sent from outside of your body. In fact most times signals and warnings of stress are coming from your own Chattering Mind. Every story in your Chattering Mind influences whether your body is resting in the parasympathetic nervous system or preparing for action in the sympathetic nervous system.

"I am so worried about my test tomorrow."

"I am glad to be home."

"I am so mad at my sister!"

"I hope I play well in the game tomorrow."

These messages create a physiological change in you body—tipping you closer towards "rest and digest" or "flight or fight."

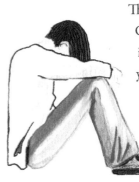

The information between your Chattering Mind and nervous system is essential to your survival. It keeps you alert and safe. As a safety feature your Chattering Mind tends to be based on self-critical, fearful, and doubting thoughts and beliefs. And these thoughts tend to loop over and over again throughout your day. Much like the looping quality of your Chattering Mind, your nervous system and brain keep looping information back and forth. So when you send a fear-based message through thought to your brain, your brain then sends information to the "flight or fight" system to kick on. When you are unaware of this process, your Chattering Mind, brain, and nervous system keep looping fear back and forth throughout your being. When this happens you begin to experience and see the world through this stressed state of your mind and body.

When you are not mindful of your own internal chatter, the above loop tends to be a default setting, to one degree or another, in all your adventures. At one end of the spectrum it leaves you constantly distracted and unable to be present to your adventure as it is miraculously unfolding. On the other end, this heightened way of living can lead to anxiety, exhaustion, obsessive thinking, and depression. However, through awareness and wise attention, there are ways to consciously work with your Chattering Mind and intelligent nervous system.

CHAPTER 3

"Thoughts are like the breeze or the leaves on the trees or the raindrops falling. They appear like that and through inquiry we can make friends with them."

—Byron Katie

Y our Inner Navigator is naturally open, spacious, and free. Think back to when you were a baby—the very first day, even, that you came into this world. You were fresh and bright and wide open to all that was happening. You had no plans, nowhere to be, and nothing pressing that you needed to do. You were fully present to all of the faces, sounds, and sensations around you. You trusted everyone completely for your warmth, food, and comfort.

In your adventure of Life, you actively acquire and learn information to function in the world. Every day, you actively learn abstract concepts like speaking, writing, and reading to communicate with others around you. You learn how to reason with your parents so that you can have your desires met. You know how to care for yourself—how and what to eat, how to use the bathroom, how to brush your teeth. Each day, you are actively gathering information about the world around you.

You also learn by watching and absorbing all around you. You notice how your mom and dad interact—their loving

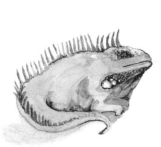
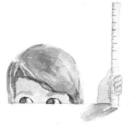

embraces, their stressors, how they treat one another when disagreeing. You are aware of how other families—moms, dads, brothers, sisters, grandparents, aunts, and uncles—interact and treat one another. You note what behavior is deemed positive by your teacher's reactions to you and your classmates. And you absorb what is acceptable and unacceptable in your local community and global community by witnessing how others act and react towards each other.

The process of gaining and storing information is necessary for your survival as a Great Adventurer. It gives you skills for survival and information for your Inner Navigator to successfully move you through your Life. Your brain is ablaze with neuron activity and pathways created by all you have learned until this point. Your Inner Navigator deeply stores this learned information from your family, culture, and society and relays it to you through your Chattering Mind.

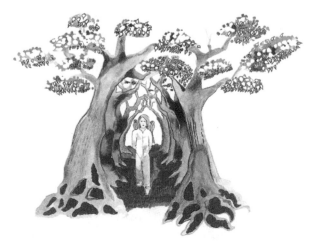

Much of this relaying happens under your conscious awareness. As you go about your day your Chattering Mind is always on the look out for your well being, pushing away what it deems unwanted and moving you towards what it finds pleasurable. Based only on past information running in a constant loop, the Chattering Mind hardly lets in any new, fresh information. This puts your Inner Navigator into an automatic, almost half-asleep mode of being—relying solely on the Chattering Mind.

Think back again to the day you were born—your wide open, fresh, free Inner Navigator. This is the original state of your Inner Navigator. This Open Mind is still within you. You still possess all the qualities of your Open Mind—an ability to be present, an ability to take in the vastness of possibilities of each moment, and an ability to have fresh, new thoughts that are not a part of the same old loop. Your Open Mind is always connected to the present moment, open to your Life as it is happening, without the influence of your Chattering Mind. It is just so covered over by all the chatter that you may have forgotten it is there.

Your Open Mind also has the mysterious ability to be aware of your Chattering Mind. When you find your Inner Attention and mindfully place it on your Chattering Mind, you begin to hear what you are saying to yourself.

And almost magically, placing your Inner Attention on your Chattering Mind begins to lessen its unconscious pull on you.

You may have had flashes of your Open Mind while in nature. It awakens when you sit at the ocean's edge, look at the grandeur of the mountains, or see the mystery of the night sky. Or maybe you have had glimpses of your Open Mind while fully absorbed in doing something you love. You connect to your Open Mind when you paint, play music, ride your bike, or score a goal in soccer.

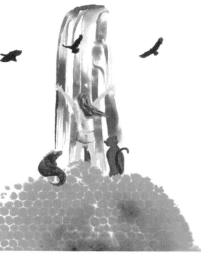

Your Open Mind's home is the present moment. You know you are seeing the world through your Open Mind when you feel fully present, enlivened by your adventure, and deeply at peace on your journey. The presence and aliveness you feel in these moments are at the core of your Open Mind.

Both your Chattering Mind and Open Mind are important parts of your Inner Navigator and each has specific skills that are necessary for your adventure. How your adventure unfolds and the quality of your adventure has a lot to do with your awareness and understanding of how each operates and relates to the other.

This, Great Adventurer, just might be the most exciting (and sometimes treacherous) part of your adventure—to look deeply into your own Chattering Mind, to know fully your Open Mind, and to have a conscious relationship between the two. Your ability to know and live from your Open Mind and consciously use your Chattering Mind as a tool will assist you more than anyone or anything else on your adventure. With this wisdom you will create the most amazing adventure this world has ever seen!

CHAPTER 4

"The past is over and the future has not yet arrived. Since the present moment is the only real moment for us, we can always return there to get in touch with the wonders of life."

—Thich Nat Hanh

Learning to live in the spaciousness of your Open Mind and seeing your Chattering Mind clearly are skills—and like learning any skill it takes lots of practice. Just as you would strengthen your physical body in preparation for a marathon with a daily practice of running, eating well, and resting, so too you need to strengthen your ability daily to see your Chattering Mind and to know your Open Mind. The skills to strengthen your connection to your Open Mind are:

- Shining the light of Awareness on both your Open Mind and Chattering Mind
- Exploring your Chattering Mind
- Wisely placing your Inner Attention in the Open Mind
- Developing a conscious relationship between your Chattering Mind and Open Mind

Let's start with Awareness. Awareness is the foundation to knowing deeply your Open Mind and your Chattering

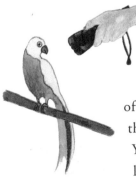

Mind. Awareness is your inner ability to open your focus and clearly see the present moment. This means taking in fully, without the obstructed view of your Chattering Mind, your own thoughts, body, and environment. You can imagine your Awareness is like a flashlight, wherever you shine

that light you are able to see more clearly, bringing the present moment into clear focus.

On one hand your Awareness is a step towards knowing and living from your Open Mind because both live in the present moment. When you use your inner flashlight, you connect to your ability to be present. On the other hand your Awareness allows you to know your Chattering Mind by always hearing what you're saying to yourself day in and day out. With your Awareness you can see how your Chattering Mind is almost never in the present moment, clouding your Inner Attention's ability to see clearly.

Once you gain strength in using your Awareness to really become conscious of two parts of the Inner Navigator—your Open Mind and Chattering Mind—you can then investigate what you say to yourself. As you begin to pay attention, be sure not to judge or ever change what your Chattering Mind is saying. You want to know your own thoughts so well— like you want to know your dearest friend. And just like you would treat your friend with love and kindness, so too you want to treat whatever you find in your Chattering Mind. You are simply paying attention.

Take the time to know your chatter deeply. Compassionately notice everything about each story in your Chattering Mind. Is this story driven by fear? False beliefs? Not deserving? Where did the story come from? Is it really true? How does my body react to this story? How does it make me feel? Remember your courage and compassion as you investigate what is in your Chattering Mind. Some wild stories may show themselves to you. Know that all Adventurers have wild, even anxious, stories. So hang on and be brave!

As you examine your Chattering Mind, stay aware of your Open Mind. Even imagine that your Open Mind is holding and patiently exploring each story your Chatting Mind spins, no matter how stormy. As you hold your Chattering Mind in your Open Mind notice the shift of your Inner Attention. Instead of unconsciously living under the influence of your Chattering Mind, you are beginning to live consciously from the presence and freedom of your Open Mind. This is BIG!

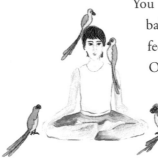

You will notice your body feels more balanced and peaceful and your heart feels more light and joyful. Your Open Mind is becoming your home base to navigate from on your wild and adventurous Life!

Where you place your Inner Attention is also an important part of your daily practice and inward shift. If your Awareness is the flashlight that illuminates what is in the present moment, then your Inner Attention is much like a magnifying glass focusing your attention on what is right in front of you. Most times your Chattering Mind clouds over your Inner Attention's ability to see what is actually happening right in front of you, seeing instead from your past experiences, likes, and dislikes.

There is the present moment and then there is what your Chattering Mind thinks of the present moment. When this happens you react from the cloud of the Chattering Mind, instead of the open reality of the present moment. Your magnifying glass keeps you connected to the reality of the moment, instead of to your stories about it.

Placing your Inner Attention may be the part that takes the most practice and therefore the most patience. Remind yourself that this is a process, and like any great skill it takes practice. Many times throughout your day, you will find your Awareness "waking up" to the fact that your Inner Attention is not present, but lost in your Chattering Mind. Don't fret! This is common to all Adventurers and a large part of your journey. This "waking up" is a gift. You remembered your Awareness and now it becomes an opportunity to practice placing your Inner Attention back in the present, back in your Open Mind. Here you can hold the stories that you find with the light of your flashlight and the clarity of your magnifying glass.

This is exciting because it gives you a choice—to either unconsciously go along with the old habits of your Chattering Mind or to wake up fully to the freshness of the present moment. Inner Attention placed in the present moment opens you to all that you are—your original, open, present Inner Navigator.

When you are present you are connected to the qualities of your heart—like love, joy, and compassion. When you are present, you can see clearly what is happening before you and make the wisest choice in that moment. When you are present, you are connected to your deep strength, power and patience—all of which help you to open bravely to whatever is, no matter how challenging or enjoyable. Your Inner Attention, placed consciously and wisely in your Open Mind, allows you to live this adventurous Life to its fullest!

All of this is not to say that your Chattering Mind is not important—it is necessary. 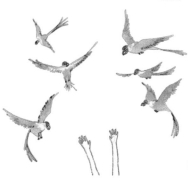 You need your Chattering Mind's ability to remember and focus, which moves you safely through your Life. Your Chattering Mind not only keeps you safe, but assists you in bringing into form all of your ideas, dreams, and goals. Your Chattering Mind can even help connect you to others by allowing you to express and share what you find in your heart. You need your Chattering Mind to navigate this adventurous Life.

The key to a healthy Chattering Mind is to always remember that it is just a tool of your Inner Navigator—a spectacular, amazing tool—but a tool nonetheless. You are not just your Chattering Mind. Your stories, your fears, your worries—even your goals, accomplishments, and desires—are just a small part of who you are. This small part is always held within the spaciousness and presence of your original, Open Mind.

Using your flashlight and magnifying glass, you can dissolve stressful, self-limiting chatter into the openness of the present moment. This is very freeing. When a story is stressful, overwhelming, or distracting you can let it go and connect to the freshness of your Open Mind. Remembering this will allow you to consciously use your Chattering Mind, instead of allowing it to swallow you.

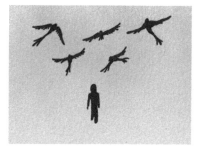

Wherever you find yourself, Great Adventurer, always remember to use your Chattering Mind consciously. Pay attention to what it is up to. Question what it is saying about you and others. Hold lovingly what you find in the clearness of your Open Mind. Wisely place your Inner Attention back in your Open Mind each time you notice it has wandered. And allow your Chattering Mind to relax into your original, Open Mind. There is no better way to throw open the doors and adventure confidently and joyously into your Great Life!

CHAPTER 5

"Silence fertilizes the deep place where personality grows. A life with a peaceful center can weather all storms."

—Norman Vincent Peale

Daily Practices

Ways to explore and know your Chattering Mind and Open Mind are as unique and varied as each person's beautiful brain. The following suggestions and practices have led many Adventurers to experience and know their Open Mind. They are meant to be guideposts along your path—not to be adhered to strictly, but used in your own creative way. A big part of your adventure will depend on your ability to open beyond the concepts of your Chattering Mind and trust what you find.

Present Moment Awareness

Your Open Mind lives in the present moment. The more you shift your attention into the present moment, the more connected you will feel to your Open Mind. The more connected you feel, the more you will trust and live from your Open Mind. Three sure-fire ways to bring your attention into the present moment are:

- Breath Awareness
- Body Awareness
- Awareness of Silence

These three exercises can be done anytime, anywhere. When you find yourself lost in your Chattering Mind or flung into your sympathetic nervous system, know these three practices are always available to you. Much like a secret weapon, no one would even know when you are using them and they are yours to use whenever you need them.

Breath Awareness

Your breath is always in the present moment. Its graceful, fluid movement is fueled by this world you are a part of—it connects you to every person, animal, and plant on the earth. Each time you inhale, you are breathing in the air that everyone before you has breathed. Each time you exhale, you are sending your breath back into the air that each of us breathes.

Every time you place your Inner Attention on your breath, you are stepping out of the unconscious Chattering Mind and towards the presence of your Open Mind. With each mindful, deep breath, your diaphragm expands through its full movement in the rib cage. This full movement of your diaphragm sends a message to your nervous system that you are safe and well. This switch sends you into your "rest and digest" mode, which then allows your brain to relax. Now you can step towards your Open Mind.

The practice of Breath Awareness is — wherever you are, when you "wake up" to the fact that you are not present and lost in your Chattering Mind, you kindly invite your Inner Attention to your breath. Follow your breath with your Inner Attention. Really experience what it feels like to breathe—the tickle of air through your nose, the expanding of your ribs fully, the feeling of release as you exhale. As you feel your breath, stay aware of the presence of your Open Mind.

Body Awareness

The sensations of your body are also happening in the present moment. Your beating heart, the feeling of your feet in your shoes on the ground, the texture of your clothes on your skin are all bridges to bring your Inner Attention out of your Chattering Mind and back into the present moment. The more you invite your Inner Attention to the sensations of your body, the more you draw your attention out of the Chattering Mind. Every movement and each sensation are an opportunity to step fully awake into your Life.

Most times when you are lost in the fog of your Chattering Mind, you start to feel like a head pulling around a body. This is disjointing for your body and starts to shift you towards your "flight or fight" mode. Consciously bringing your Inner Attention into the fullness of your physical body calms your brain and allows you to feel more whole and alive. Instead of just a head, you are an embodied and present Adventurer.

The practice of Body Awareness is — when you "wake up" to the fact that you are not present and are lost in your Chattering Mind, kindly invite your Inner Attention to the feeling of your whole body. Feel your feet in your shoes placed firmly on the ground. Feel the wind and sun on your skin. Feel the sensation of your palms resting on your legs. As you experience the feeling of your body, stay aware of the presence of your Open Mind.

Awareness of Silence

Your Chattering Mind is a loud and active place most days. And the more your Chattering Mind is stimulated by television, computers, smart phones, video games, and music, the louder your Chattering Mind becomes. Your Chattering Mind thrives on entertainment and distraction. It loves to be occupied by all the noise of our technological world and stimulated by everything you see and hear.

But underneath all the noise of our technological world and the Chattering Mind is a ground of silence. You can hear it when you switch off all your electronic devices and allow your Inner Attention to step out of your inner dialogue and into the spacious clarity of the quiet. You can even see how the natural world seems to live in this silence. The warm afternoon sun silently shining on your favorite tree. The wild flowers growing quietly in the meadow. The stars moving across the vastness of the open sky. This quiet is empty of all of your stories about who you are or who you think you should be. It is open to all of the possibilities of who you are and can be.

The practice of Awareness of Silence is — when you notice you are lost in the fog of your Chattering Mind, kindly invite your inner attention out of your Chatter and into the silence around you. If you need to unplug everything, go for it! You may even need to get outside to a quiet spot under a tree. As you shift your inner attention to silence, stay aware of the presence of your Open Mind.

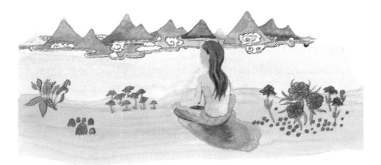

You were born free and open. This is who you truly are, Great Adventurer. You are not the chatter. You are alive with the full potential of the present moment. You were born completely whole with everything you need. This compete wholeness is still with you. If you pay attention you can hear it gently calling to you, inviting you to remember, every step of your journey.

May you step bravely and joyfully into your wholeness and Open Mind. May each brave step bring you the Adventure of a Life fully and joyfully lived!

REBECCA BRENNER is an author, teacher, speaker, and practitioner of the integrative healing arts. She holds a Ph.D. in nutrition and is a certified yoga and meditation teacher through the Himalayan Institute and the Sivananda Yoga Vedanta Centers. She leads popular wellness, yoga, and mindfulness classes in Park City, Utah and works individually with clients and families through her consulting practice, Park City Holistic Health. A mother of two girls, she is passionate about sharing how to live a healthy human life with just about anyone who will listen.

BROOKE KEMMERER is a freelance illustrator and artist living in Jackson, Wyoming. She received her BFA from the School of the Art Institute of Chicago in 2006, and an MA in Spiritual Psychology from the University of Santa Monica in 2010. A lover of eastern philosophy Brooke has spent her years traveling through Asia and studying Tibetan Buddhism and Thangka painting. She is a mother of a two-year-old named Stella, and her newborn son Locke. Brooke enjoys balancing her fairly new role as mother with her passion for painting and love of the outdoors.

For more information or to connect with the Kid's User Guide community, visit us at www.facebook.com/KidsUserGuide or http://kidsuserguide.wordpress.com. Stay tuned for The Kid's User Guide to a Human Life Book Two.

CPSIA information can be obtained at www.ICGtesting.com
Printed in the USA
BVOW10s1405051114

373811BV00007B/11/P

9 781614 489238